Invigorating Sugar Scrub Recipes

By
Gene Ashburner

ISBN-13:978-1503083820
ISBN-10:1503083829

Content

Almond Sugar Scrub

Ingredients

500 ml white sugar

125 ml almond oil

125 ml almond milk

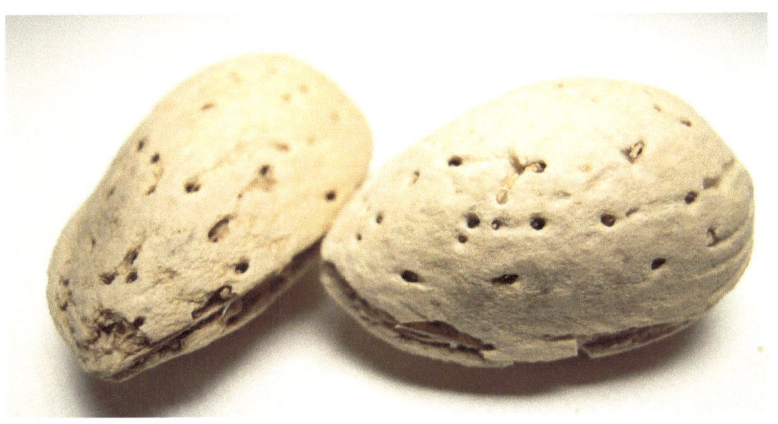

Method

Combine all the ingredients together.

Mix well.

Apple Cinnamon Sugar Scrub

Ingredients

500 ml brown sugar

250 ml almond oil

10 ml ground cinnamon

8 drops apple aromatherapy oil

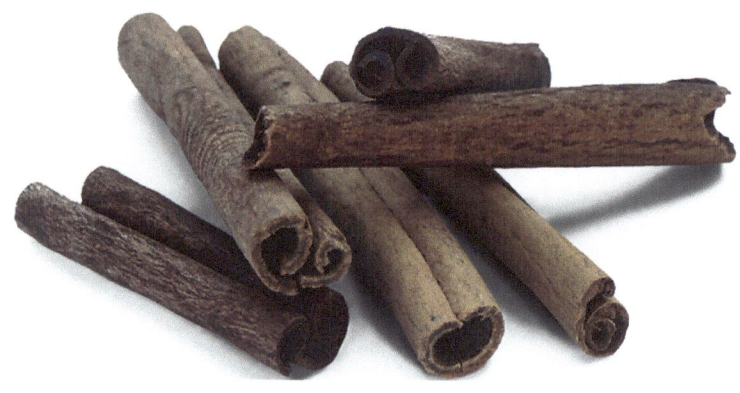

Method

Combine all the ingredients together.

Mix well.

Apricot Sugar Scrub

Ingredients

500 ml brown sugar
250 ml apricot kernel oil
8 drops apricot essential oil

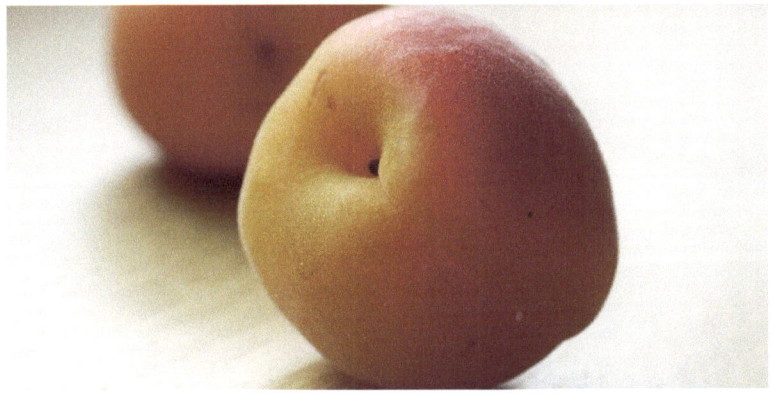

Method

Combine all the ingredients together.
Mix well.

Avocado Sugar Scrub

Ingredients

2 avocados (peeled and stoned)
25 ml lemon juice
250 ml apricot kernel oil
25 ml pure honey
500 ml sugar

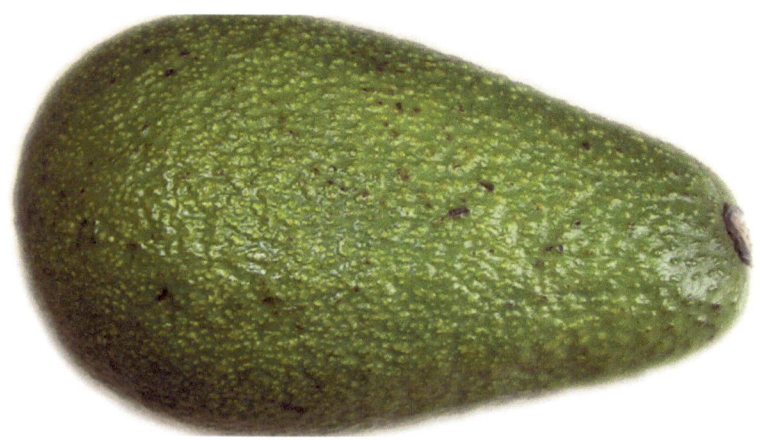

Method

Blend the avocados, lemon juice, apricot kernel oil and honey together in a food blender.

Blend until smooth.

Remove from blender.

Add the sugar.

Mix well.

Apricot Sugar Scrub

Ingredients

500 ml brown sugar

250 ml apricot kernel oil

8 drops apricot essential oil

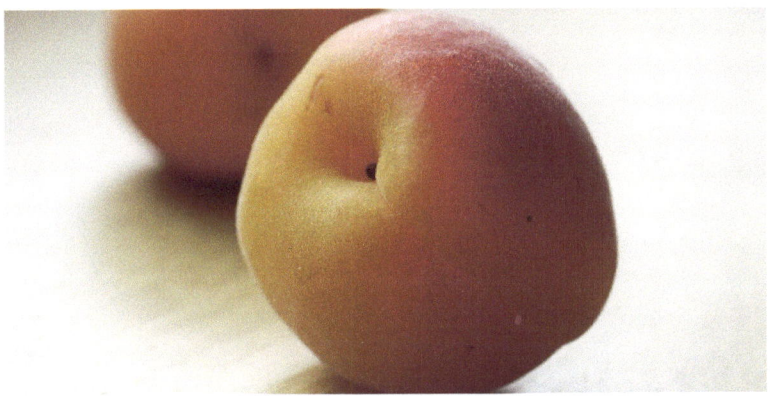

Method

Combine all the ingredients together.

Mix well.

Avocado Sugar Scrub

Ingredients

2 avocados (peeled and stoned)
25 ml lemon juice
250 ml apricot kernel oil
25 ml pure honey
500 ml sugar

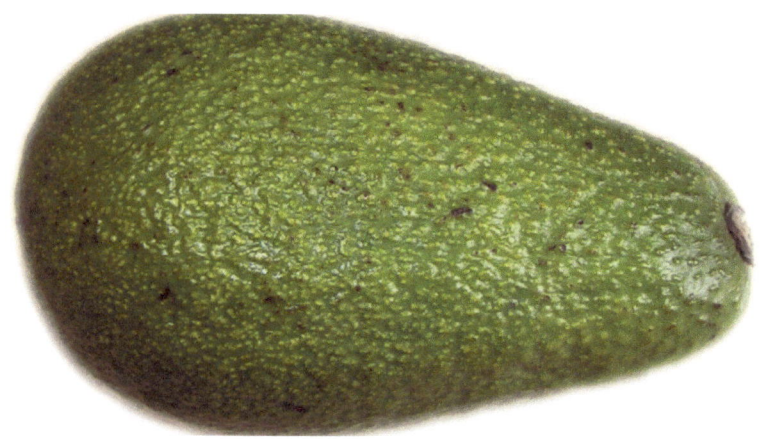

Method

Blend the avocados, lemon juice, apricot kernel oil and honey together in a food blender.

Blend until smooth.

Remove from blender.

Add the sugar.

Mix well.

Basil And Lime Sugar Scrub

Ingredients

500 ml white sugar

250 ml almond oil

5 drops lime essential oil

4 drops basil oil

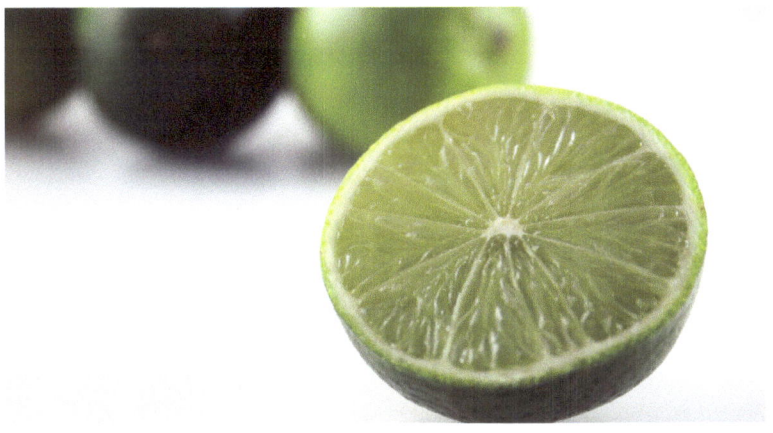

Method

Combine all the ingredients together.

Mix well.

Brown Sugar Rose Scrub

Ingredients

500 ml dark brown sugar

250 ml almond oil

10 ml pure rose water

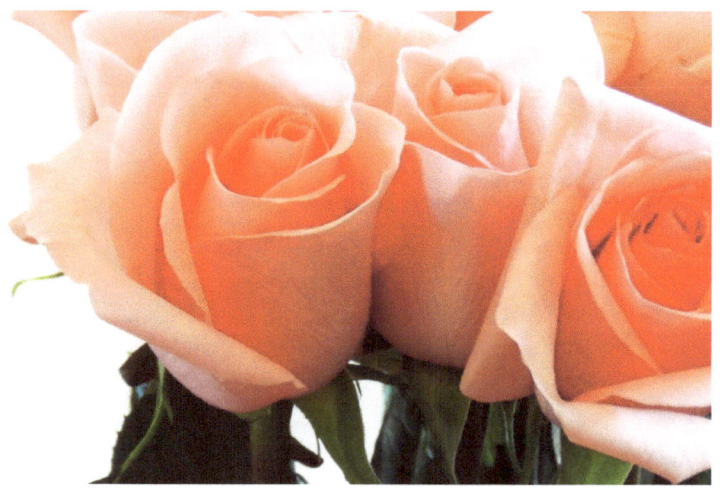

Method

Combine all the ingredients together.

Mix well.

Brown Sugar Scrub

Ingredients

500 ml dark brown sugar

250 ml almond oil

10 ml pure vanilla extract

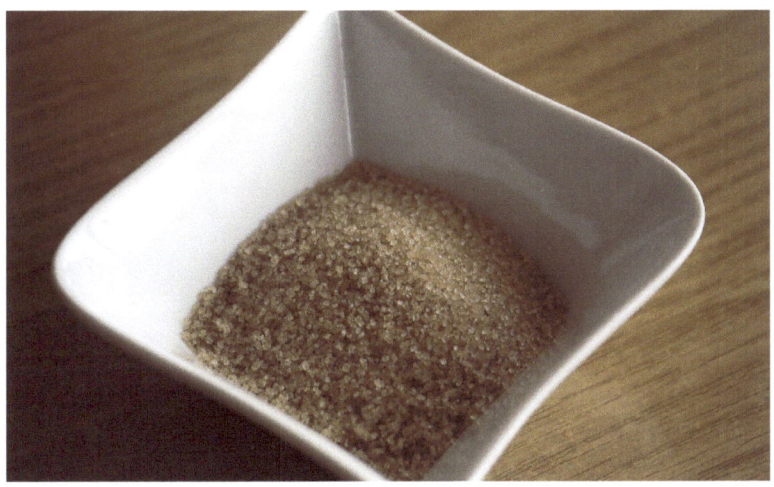

Method

Combine all the ingredients together.

Mix well.

Cherry Almond Sugar Scrub

Ingredients

500 ml white sugar

250 ml almond oil

5 drops cherry aromatherapy oil

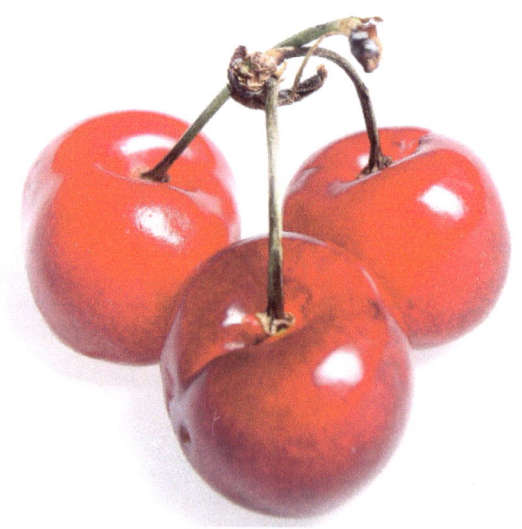

Method

Combine all the ingredients together.

Mix well.

Chocolate Hazelnut Sugar Scrub

Ingredients

500 ml sugar

250 ml hazelnut oil

5 ml chocolate fragrance oil

10 ml cocoa powder

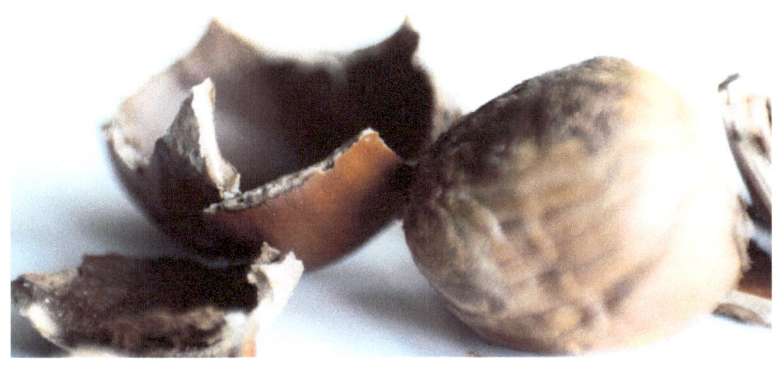

Method

Combine all the ingredients together.

Mix well.

Cinnamon Sugar Scrub

Ingredients

500 ml brown sugar
250 ml almond oil
10 ml ground cinnamon

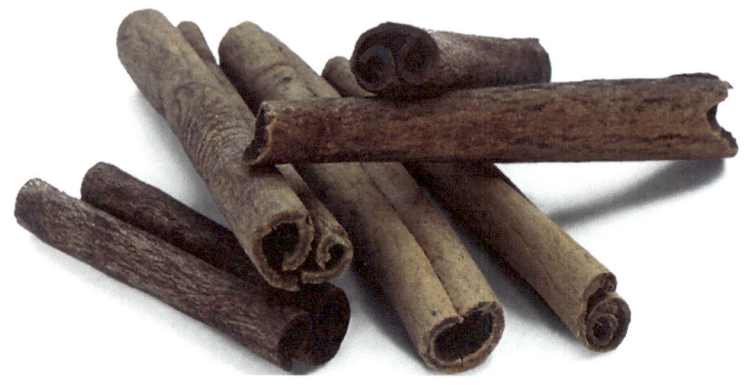

Method

Combine all the ingredients together.
Mix well.

Coconut Sugar Scrub

Ingredients

500 ml sugar

250 ml coconut oil

25 ml shredded coconut

5 ml coconut fragrance oil

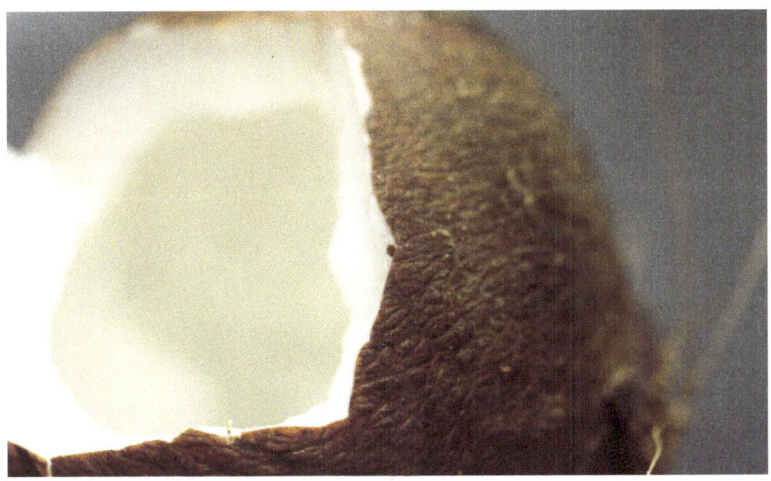

Method

Combine all the ingredients together.

Mix well.

Coffee Sugar Scrub

Ingredients

500 ml brown sugar
250 ml jojoba oil
10 ml coffee powder

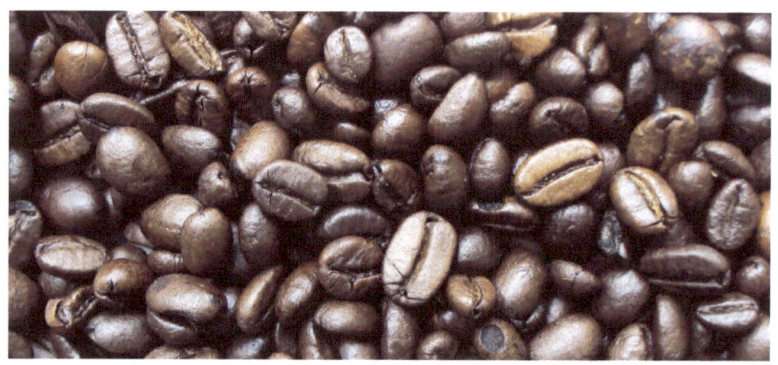

Method

Combine all the ingredients together.
Mix well.

Ginger Sugar Scrub

Ingredients

500 ml white sugar

125 ml coconut oil

125 ml almond oil

10 ml ground ginger

5 drops lemongrass essential oil

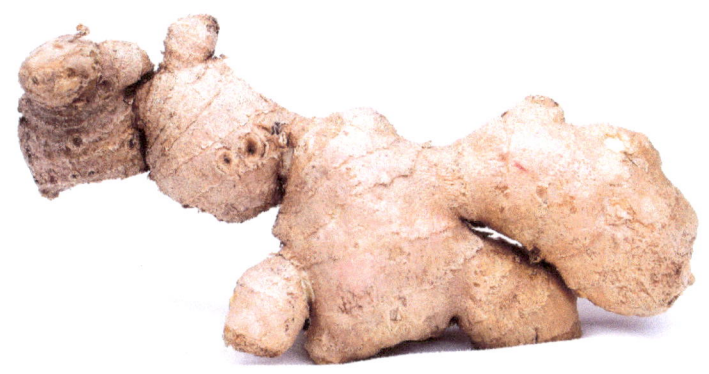

Method

Combine all the ingredients together.

Mix well.

Grapefruit Sugar Scrub

Ingredients

375 ml white sugar

125 ml jojoba oil

12,5 ml grapefruit essential oil

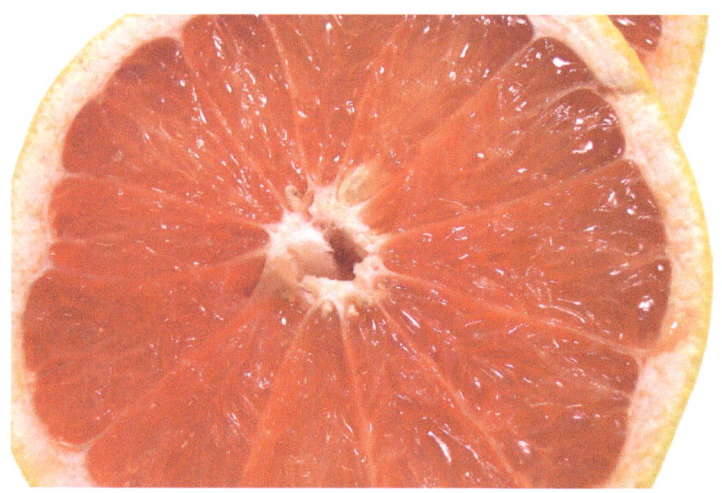

Method

Combine all the ingredients together.

Mix well.

Herb Sugar Scrub

Ingredients

500 ml dark brown sugar

250 ml olive oil

5 drops rosemary oil

5 drops sage oil

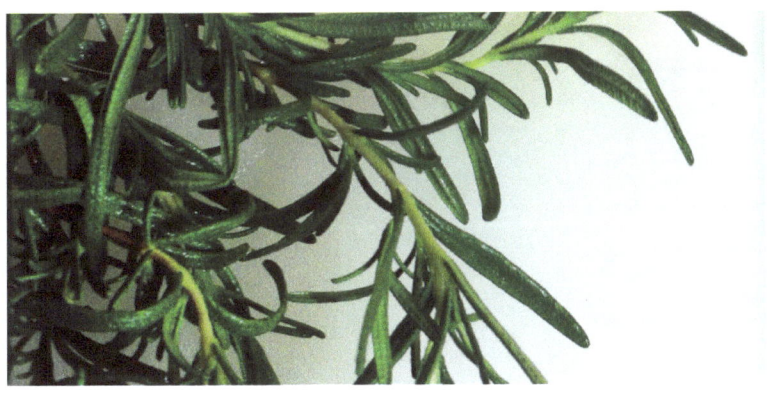

Method

Combine all the ingredients together.

Mix well.

Hibiscus Geranium Sugar Scrub

Ingredients

500 ml white sugar

125 ml almond oil

125 ml apricot kernel oil

12,5 ml hibiscus flower powder

5 drops geranium essential oil

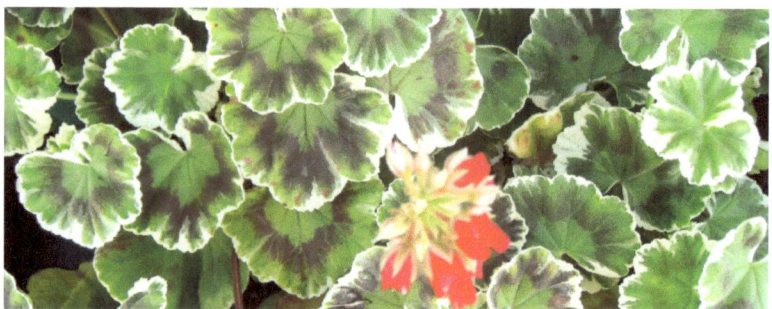

Method

Combine all the ingredients together.

Mix well.

Hibiscus Ginger Sugar Scrub

Ingredients

500 ml white sugar

250 ml olive oil

12,5 ml hibiscus flower powder

5 drops ginger and orange essential oil

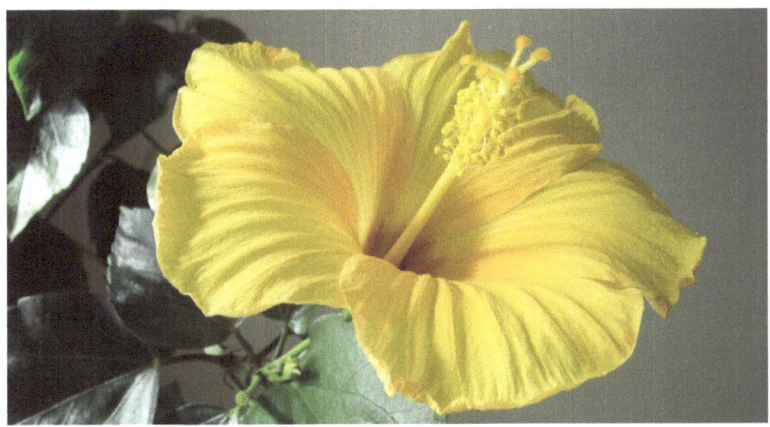

Method

Combine all the ingredients together.

Mix well.

Hibiscus Rose Sugar Scrub

Ingredients

500 ml white sugar

250 ml almond oil

12,5 ml hibiscus flower powder

5 drops rose essential oil

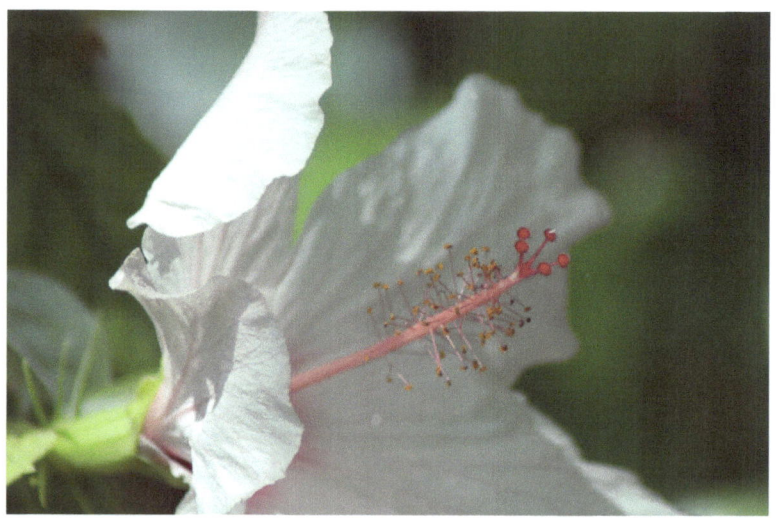

Method

Combine all the ingredients together.

Mix well.

Honey Almond Sugar Scrub

Ingredients

375 ml white sugar

125 ml honey

10 ml almond extract

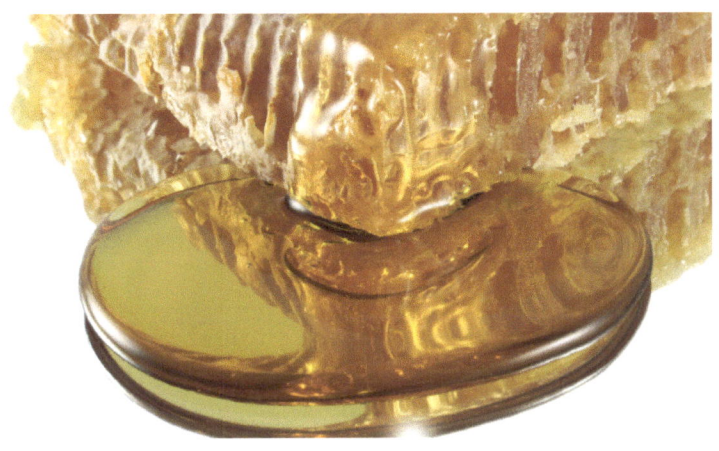

Method

Combine all the ingredients together.

Mix well.

Honey Pistachio Sugar Scrub

Ingredients

500 ml white sugar

125 ml honey

125 ml pistachio oil

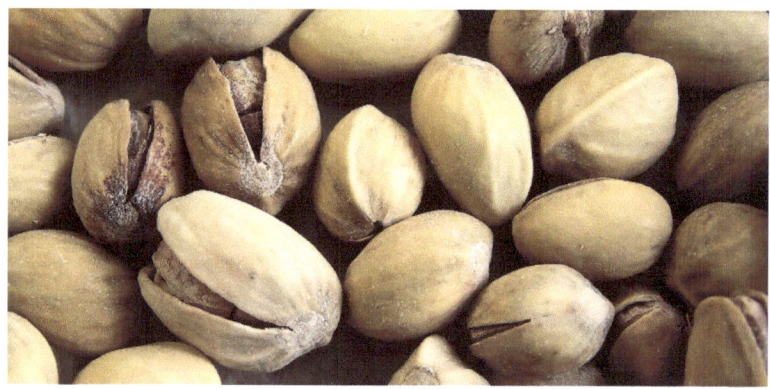

Method

Combine all the ingredients together.

Mix well.

Jojoba Cleansing Sugar Scrub

Ingredients

500 ml white sugar

250 ml jojoba oil

5 ml essential orange oil

250 ml liquid soap

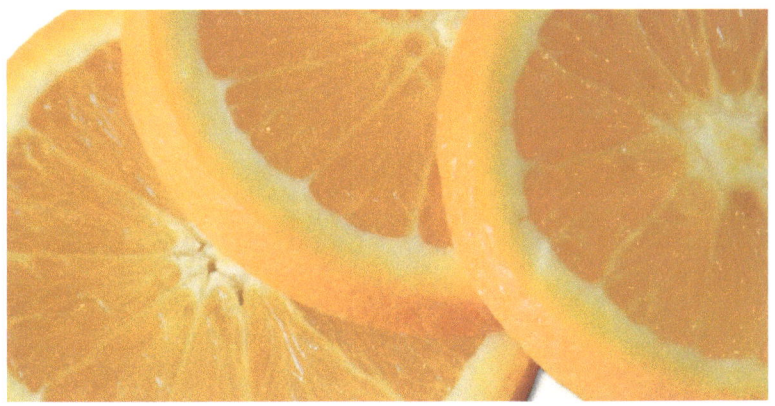

Method

Combine all the ingredients together.

Mix well.

Lavender Orange Sugar Scrub

Ingredients

500 ml white sugar

500 ml avocado oil

4 drops lavender essential oil

3 drops orange essential oil

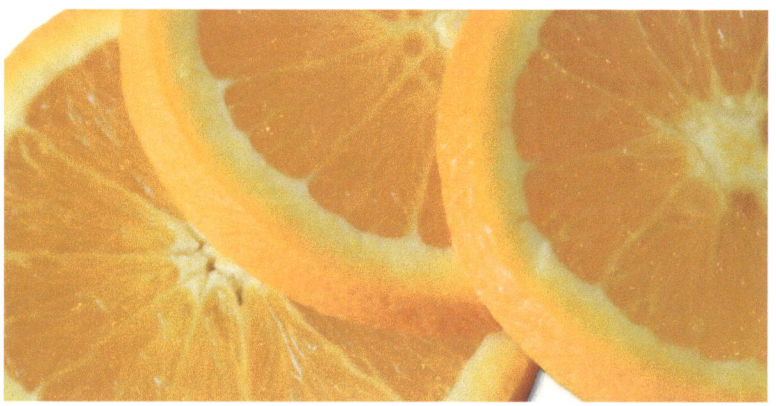

Method

Combine all the ingredients together.

Mix well.

Lavender Sugar Scrub

Ingredients

125 ml coconut oil
125 ml grape seed oil
250 ml white sugar
5 drops lavender essential oil

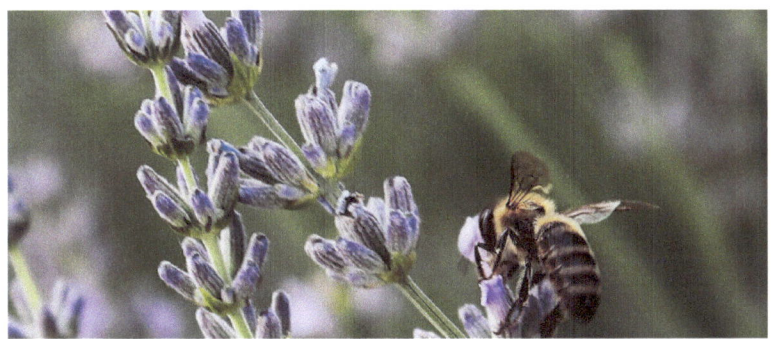

Method

Combine all the ingredients together.
Mix well.

Lemongrass Sugar Scrub

Ingredients

500 ml white sugar

250 ml olive oil

8 drops lemongrass essential oil

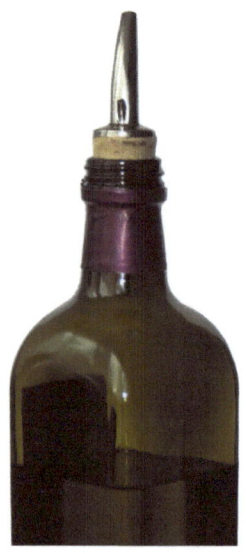

Method

Combine all the ingredients together.

Mix well.

Lemon Almond Sugar Scrub

Ingredients

500 ml sugar
50 ml almond oil
100 ml lemon juice
10 ml lemon zest

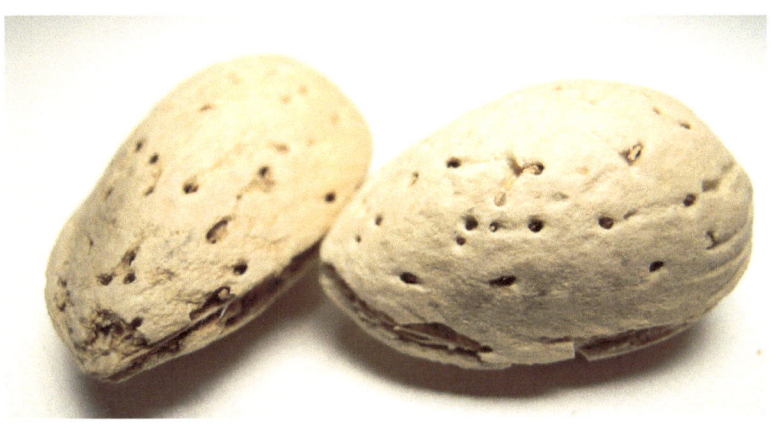

Method

Combine all the ingredients together.
Mix well.

Lemon Poppy Seed Sugar Scrub

Ingredients

500 ml sugar
50 ml almond oil
100 ml lemon juice
25 ml poppy seeds

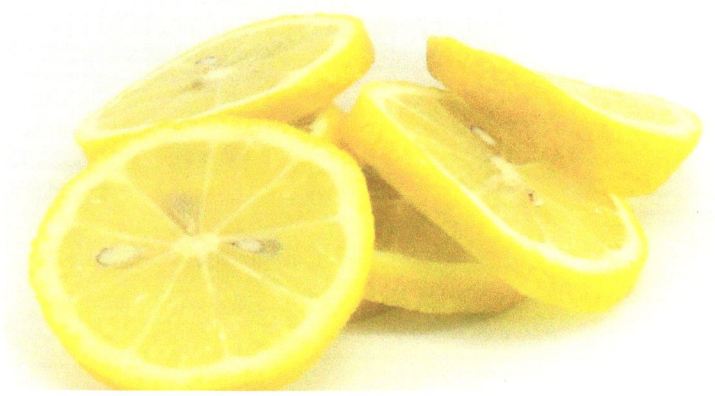

Method

Combine all the ingredients together.
Mix well.

Lime Coconut Sugar Scrub

Ingredients

250 ml sugar

250 ml coconut oil

5 drops lime essential oil

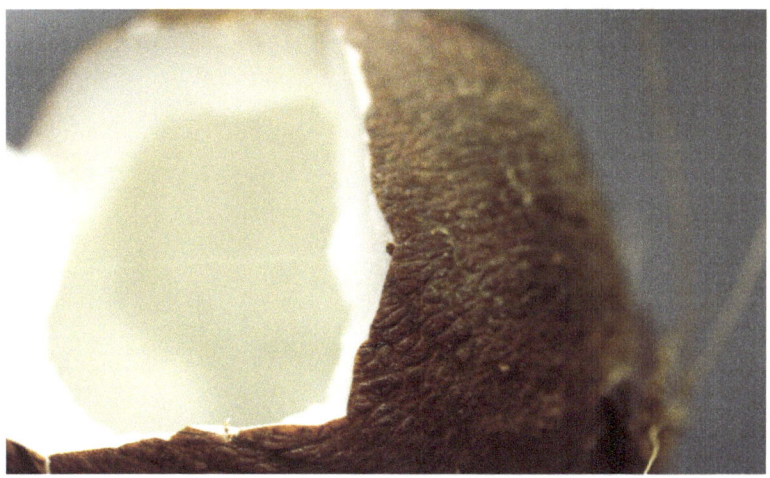

Method

Combine all the ingredients together.

Mix well.

Mango Papaya Sugar Scrub

Ingredients

1 mango (peeled, stoned and sliced)
1 papaya (peeled, seeded and sliced)
500 ml white sugar
50 ml apricot kernel oil
12,5 ml mango fragrance oil
125 ml powdered oats

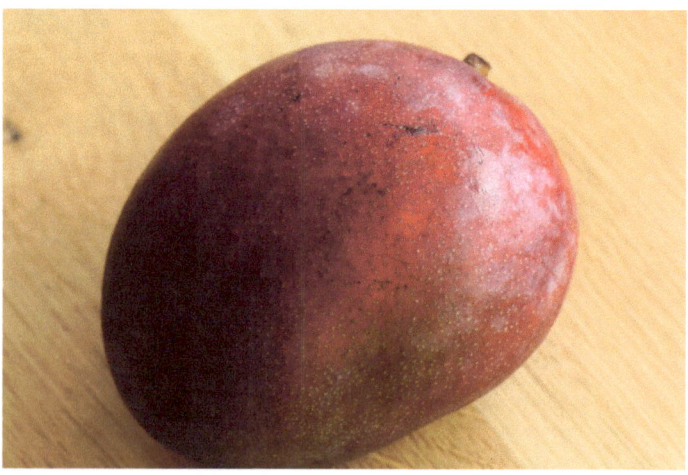

Method

Blend the mango and the papaya in a blender until almost smooth.

Combine all the ingredients together.

Mix well.

Milk Sugar Scrub

Ingredients

500 ml sugar
125 ml almond oil
125 ml whole milk

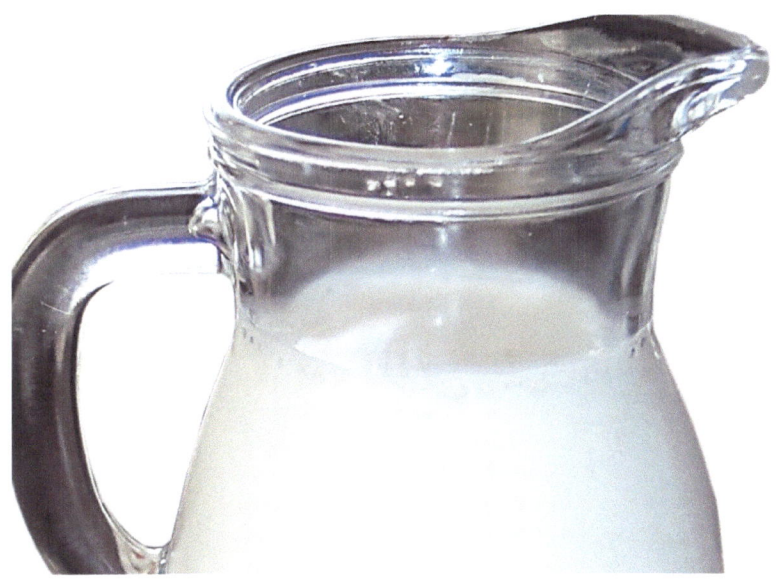

Method

Combine all the ingredients together.
Mix well.

Mocha Sugar Scrub

Ingredients

500 ml brown sugar

250 ml almond oil

50 ml ground coffee

50 ml cocoa powder

10 ml ground cinnamon

3 ml ground nutmeg

5 ml ground ginger

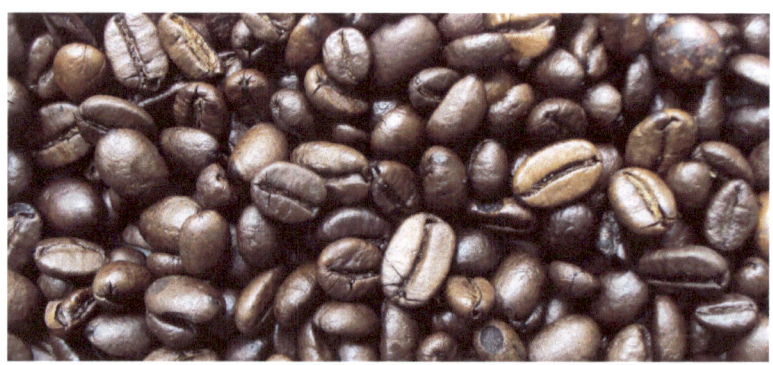

Method

Combine all the ingredients together.
Mix well.

Orange Almond Sugar Scrub

Ingredients

250 ml almond oil

250 ml white sugar

5 drops orange essential oil

10 ml orange zest

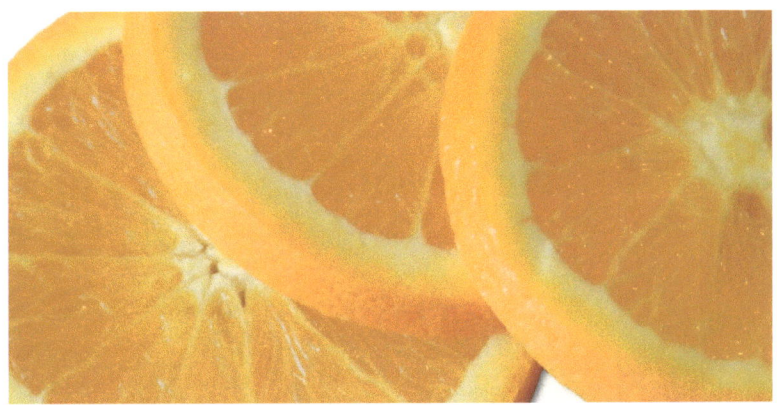

Method

Combine all the ingredients together.

Mix well.

Orange Poppy Seed Sugar Scrub

Ingredients

250 ml brown sugar

250 ml poppy seeds

250 ml olive oil

8 drops orange essential oil

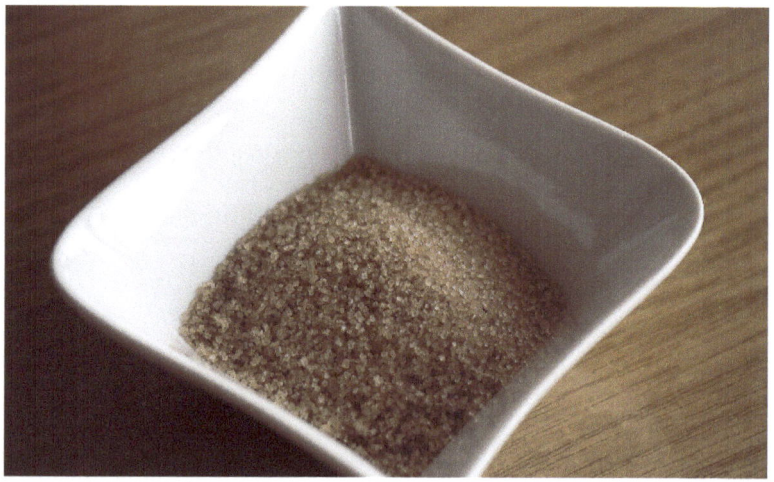

Method

Combine all the ingredients together.

Mix well.

Orange Sugar Scrub

Ingredients

500 ml brown sugar

250 ml jojoba oil

25 ml essential orange oil

3 Vitamin E capsules

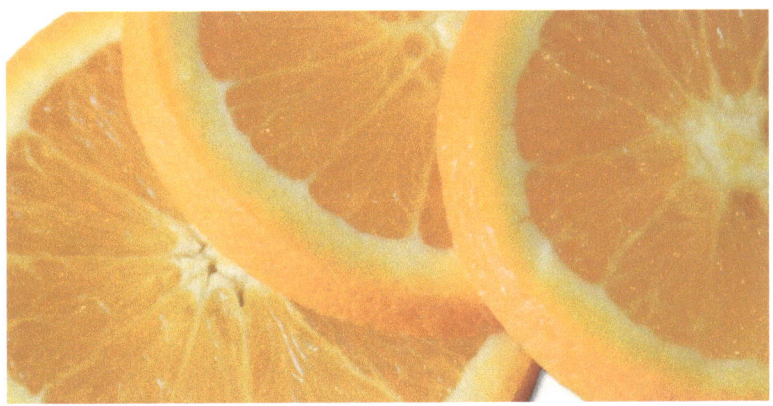

Method

Combine all the ingredients together.

Mix well.

Peach Sugar Scrub

Ingredients

500 ml white sugar

250 ml almond oil

8 drops peach aromatherapy oil

Few drops peach soap colorant

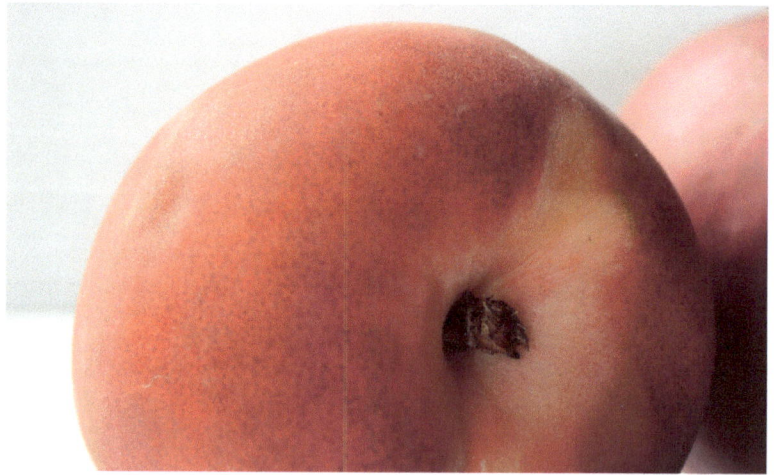

Method

Combine all the ingredients together.
Mix well.

Peppermint Sugar Scrub

Ingredients

500 ml white sugar
250 ml almond oil
8 drops peppermint essential oil

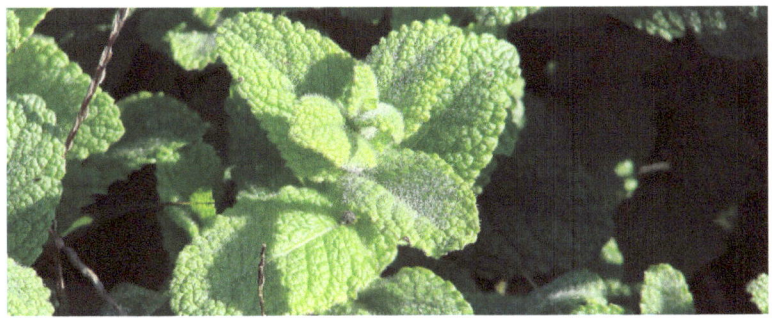

Method

Combine all the ingredients together.
Mix well.

Pineapple Coconut Sugar Scrub

Ingredients

500 ml white sugar
250 ml coconut oil
8 drops pineapple oil

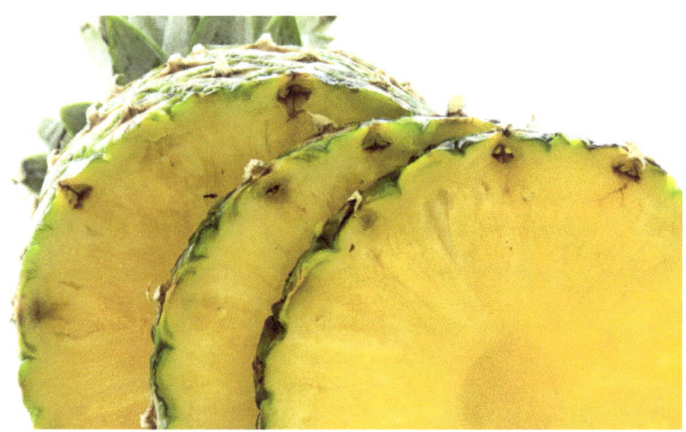

Method

Combine all the ingredients together.
Mix well.

Pistachio Rose Sugar Scrub

Ingredients

500 ml white sugar

62,5 ml pistachio oil

5 drops rose essential oil

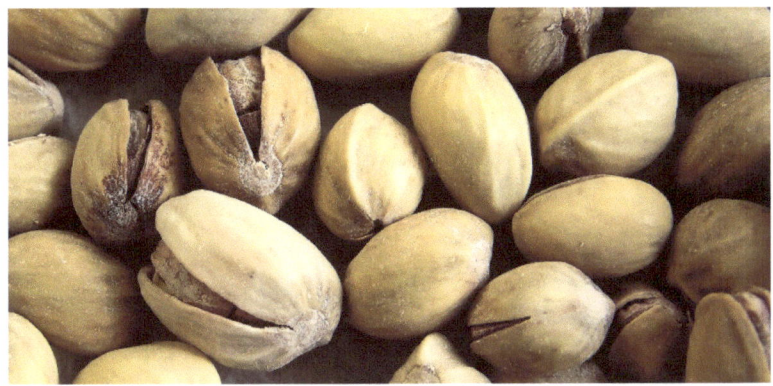

Method

Combine all the ingredients together.

Mix well.

Raspberry Sugar Scrub

Ingredients

500 ml white sugar
250 ml olive oil
8 drops raspberry oil

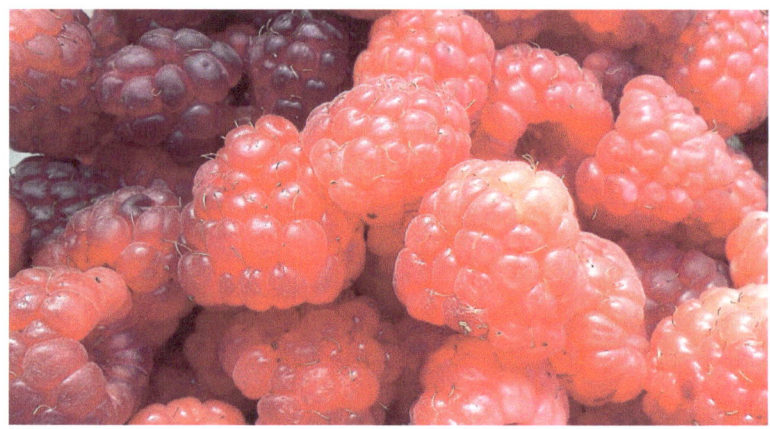

Method

Combine all the ingredients together.
Mix well.

Rosemary Sugar Scrub

Ingredients

500 ml sugar

250 ml Evening Primrose oil

3 ml Vitamin E Oil

5 drops Rosemary essential oil

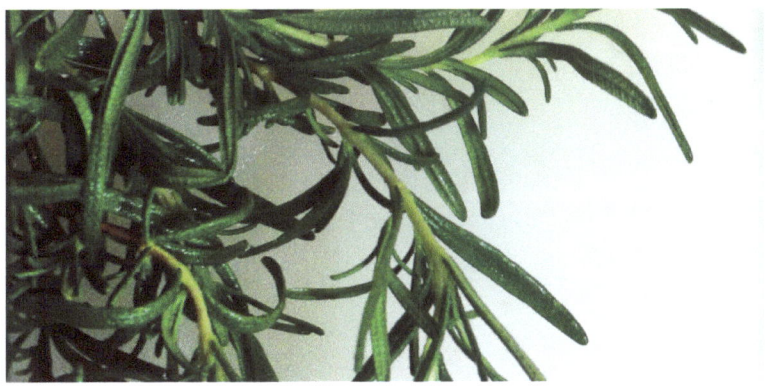

Method

Combine all the ingredients together.

Mix well.

Rose Sugar Scrub

Ingredients

125 ml coconut oil

125 ml grape seed oil

250 ml white sugar

5 drops rose essential oil

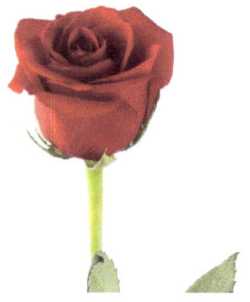

Method

Combine all the ingredients together.

Mix well.

Spicy Sugar Scrub

Ingredients

750 ml brown sugar

280 ml hazelnut oil

15 ml ground cinnamon

15 ml ground ginger

15 ml ground nutmeg

10 ml ground cardamom

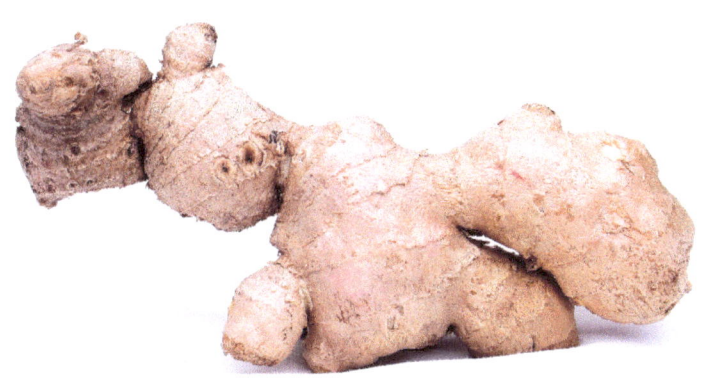

Method

Combine all the ingredients together.
Mix well.

Strawberry Sugar Scrub

Ingredients

500 ml white sugar

250 ml coconut oil

5 drops strawberry essential oil

Few drops red soap colorant

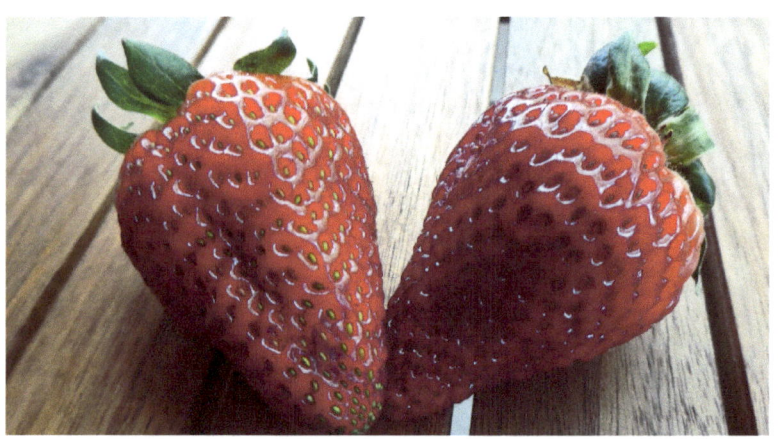

Method

Combine all the ingredients together.

Mix well.

Tangerine Sugar Scrub

Ingredients

375 ml white sugar

125 ml jojoba oil

8 ml drops tangerine essential oil

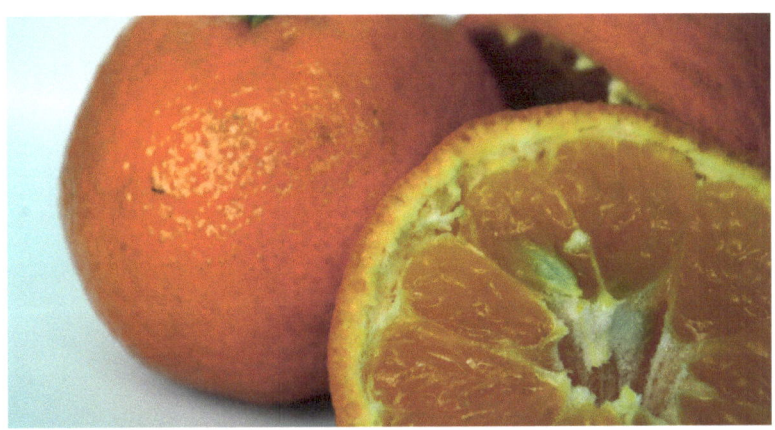

Method

Combine all the ingredients together.

Mix well.

Vanilla Brown Sugar Scrub

Ingredients

375 ml brown sugar

375 ml white sugar

375 ml olive oil

18 ml pure vanilla extract

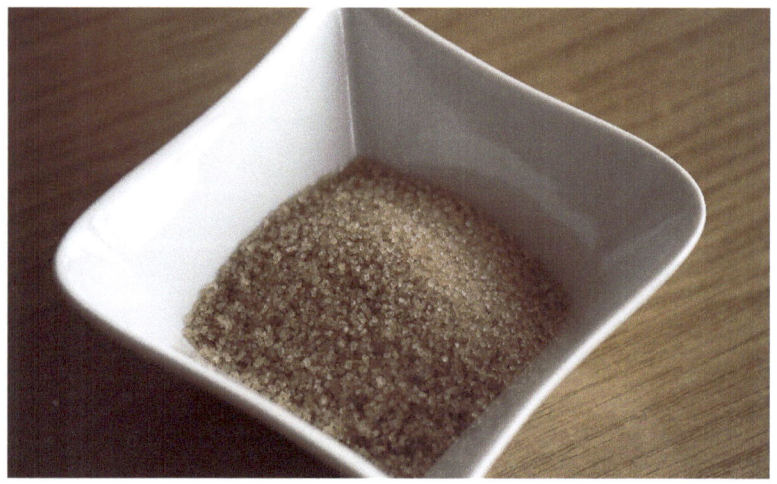

Method

Combine all the ingredients together.
Mix well.

White Chocolate Cranberry Sugar Scrub

Ingredients

500 ml sugar

4 oz cocoa butter

2 oz cranberry seed oil

Few drops (5 to 6) cranberry essential oil

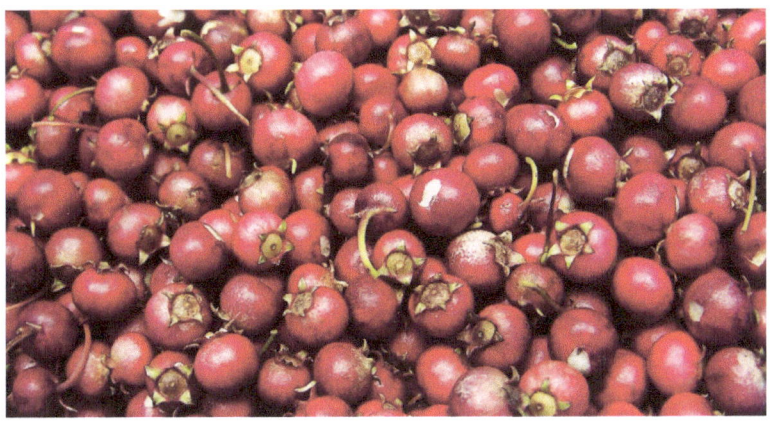

Method

Combine all the ingredients together.

Mix well.

White Chocolate Orange Sugar Scrub

Ingredients

500 ml sugar

4 oz cocoa butter

2 oz almond oil

Few drops (5 to 6) orange essential oil

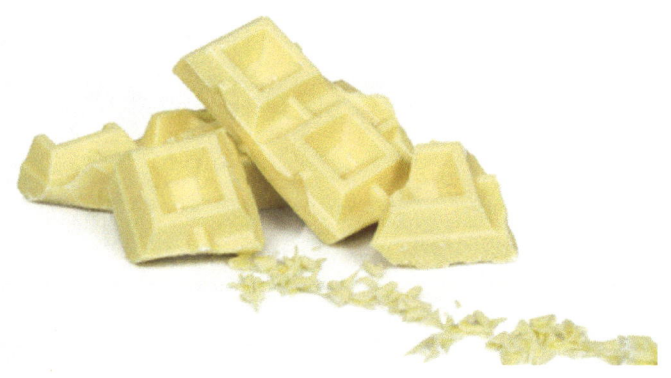

Method

Combine all the ingredients together.

Mix well.

Yogurt Sugar Scrub

Ingredients

300 ml white sugar

240 ml yogurt

200 ml brewers yeast

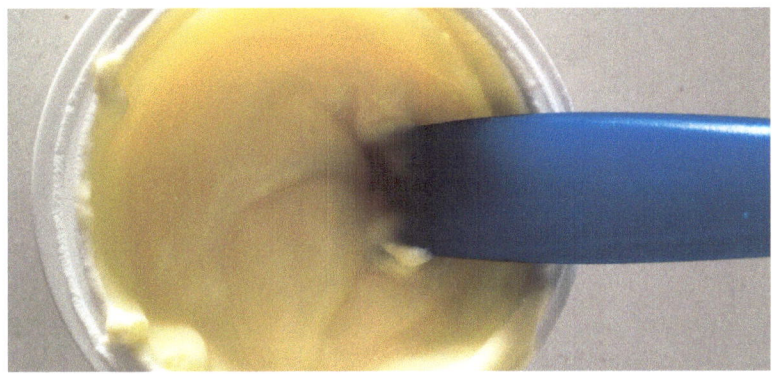

Method

Combine all the ingredients together.

Mix well.